Contents

INTRODUCTION 5

CHAPTER 1-WHAT DRIVES US 16

CHAPTER 2 THE DIFFERENCE BETWEEN FEAR &
ANXIETY 38

CHAPTER 3 - DEFINING STRESS AND THE STRESS
RESPONSE 57

CHAPTER 4 – FEAR, ANXIETY & STRESS............. 85

CHAPTER 5 – THOUGHTS, EMOTIONS,& ACTIONS
.... 114

CHAPTER 6 – WHAT KIND OF PERSONALITY ARE
YOU 154

CHAPTER 7 - COPING WITH STRESS, ANXIETY &
FEAR 175

CHAPTER EIGHT – NEGATIVE & POSITIVE COPING
TOOLS 193

DEDICATION
To the stressed, anxious and fearful

COPYRIGHT INFORMATION

Some material cited from the DSM 5 (2013) American Psychiatric Association (2013): Diagnostic and Statistical Manual of Mental Disorders (5th Ed.). Washington, DC.

Disclaimer: Material in this book are not meant for diagnosis or treatment of any disorder. It is an informational guide and not a replacement for diagnosis by a qualified mental health professional.

ISBN: 10: 1546324224
ISBN-13: 978-1546324225

INTRODUCTION

The one thing we all share in common is that we are always on the move in life; we just can't sit still for a moment to reflect or relax.

Even when we take time off from work, or our ever day life and go on a vacation it's all about the planning, trying to fit all our plans into that three or five days, in order to relax, when in reality we're still running around and not really relaxing.

However, in all this activity, even though we are supposed to be relaxing, taking it easy, we are still contributing to the ultimate problem. That is that we are stressed out, anxious and most often fearful

INTRODUCTION

just about all the time no matter where we are.

It seems to us that if we just stop for a moment something won't get done, or we'll be missing something or worse the world will end without us.

We want to "Get away from it all", but get away from what? Asked that question and people will say, "Well the job, the rush, the daily responsibilities.", and we go on a vacation and for a while, we may feel the release, but before long, we are back again worrying about how much time we got left before we return to the "same old crap".

Even when we get away, we find that what we think is the problem has somehow followed us.

INTRODUCTION

The main reason we can't seem to "shut off" the stress, anxiety and fear is because we don't understand the root of the existence. That root is contained in us, not in the things we think that if they just disappear we'll be fine.

However, that doesn't happen, indeed it can't. Even if we got onto a spaceship and went to Mars, sooner or later we would see they didn't go away.

When I teach this subject I have a saying and that is, "It's not what is without (outside), but what is within (inside). In other words, it's not the people, places and things we have to interact with in life, but what is within us that what concerns us.

INTRODUCTION

We get that completely backward. When we are asked, why we are in such a hurry, unable to relax, we will blame the "pressure", that we are under. In other words, it's because we are so stressed.

We will give a laundry list of the reasons we have so much stress. When asked about the sources of our stress, anxiety or fear, we will cite pretty much all the same reasons.

Sometimes it's the job or our boss. We stress, fear and have anxiety of how our day will go. We stress fear and have anxiety for our children, for our health, for the future, or even for the past - whether or not it will catch up with us, and on and on.

It's most likely why the sleeping aid business is a billion dollar business, helping those who suffer fear and anxiety, get some sleep. We can't sleep or eat, and when we do sleep, it is fitful, while we eat more junk food than healthy food.

Either sometimes we use excessive alcohol, prescribed or illicit drugs, smoke, to try to cope with the pressures of life.

"Yeah, it's that damn stress in my life! If you had the stress I had you'd have anxiety and fear too, and all the problems that go with it!"

Well, I understand, but from the outset, and this is the theme that I'll remind you of throughout this

---

book, and its:

"It's not what's without, it's what is within".

It's the within that we talk about in this book. This book; Mac's Guide to Coping with Stress, Anxiety, and Fear, is all about that dealing with them all, but from the INSIDE. If stress, anxiety, and fear are kicking your butt on a daily basis then you've come to the right place to get a handle on that.

How do I know that? Because they all used to thread my existence. In fact, I can't remember a time in my life when I wasn't at some time stressed out, fearful, or full of anxiety about something happening in my life, or that was going to happen or something

I did before.

However, I got a handle on it and I'll show you how it did it.

"How is that?" you might ask, and mean how I am going to teach you about stress, anxiety, and fear when I admitted to you that I've experienced them my whole life. Well, I still experience stress, anxiety, and fear, but I've gotten a lot better at not letting them rule my life.

My recovery from them began in the late 90s. In 1999, my wife was discovered to have what would be the beginning of a 14-year battle with colorectal cancer. Just months after her surgery, my mother was diagnosed with terminal lung cancer and died later that year.

Prior to that, I can't remember any significant sickness in my family, and now that idea was shattered. At the time, I was a 911 Dispatcher, one of the most stressful jobs in the world, and I began to break down under the pressure of working shifts, helping my father deal with my mom's death, and caring for my wife at the same time. It was a lot.

Then in 2000, I had a heart attack, which was strange to me seeing how at the time I jogged every day and rode a bike 40 miles a week. I was a real exercise buff. However, there I was in the emergency room, with Nitro patches on. I remember staring at a heart monitoring machine, wondering how in the heck this happened.

When the emergency room physician came in, he saw me still dressed in my running gear, and after talking with me a bit asked me to describe how life was going at the time. After I finished he told me that I was simply burned out, overwhelmed and that I should seek some help with stress management.

Well, I've never been one for that, I'm more of a self-study, so I got some books on stress, went back to college and studied psychology and began to learn about what happened to me.

What I learned not only helped me but also turned

into a Stress Management Seminar for 911 Dispatchers based what I learned and experienced on the job.

In that seminar, I covered stress, anxiety, and fear, which is a large part of the job of a 911 dispatcher, especially because the stress was mainly fear and anxiety based on fear of losing the job, fear of screwing up to the point that someone gets hurt. The seminars were a great success and I taught 911 dispatchers all over the US for over 10-years.

Then in 2009, my wife's cancer had progressed to a terminal stage, and if that weren't enough, I was too diagnosed with cancer. My wife passed away with me at her side, while I pulled through. However, during that experience, I was thankful to know what I know and use what I had learned to help me cope, and which I still use now in my daily life, lessons I know can help others.

My hope in writing this book on Coping with Stress, Anxiety, and Fear, is to help you come to terms with them in your own life, and as well cope with them positively and effectively.

Let's begin.

CHAPTER 1-WHAT DRIVES US

As I said in the introduction, one thing we all share is that we're all restless, driven, and always about finding the next best thing to make us happy.

However, does it work? I mean, if we think about it, are we all ever really happy, I mean completely happy.

If you're like most of us, you'll lower your head and say, "Not really." Why is that? Well for one, it's because everything in our world tells us that we're just not good enough, we just don't measure up.

Just look at how many books, TV and magazine ads, and other media that tell us how "incomplete" we are without this, that, and the other thing we don't have. We don't have enough money, we aren't skinny enough, our car is good enough, our house isn't big enough, and the weather isn't comfortable (too hot/too cold) enough.

We have been conditioned into this way of thinking over many, many years by various sources, but again I think it's a matter of human nature.

As an example, just look at the history of the development of The United States. People arrived on the east coast, but that wasn't good enough so we moved out west searching until we got to California and couldn't expand any further and discovered that being there wasn't good enough either.

I think that's why Californians are so "earthy" and meditative, because failing to reach peace externally, they began to look inward.

Yet in reality, our fear and anxiety drive this in all of us, mainly of not reaching our potential – whatever that is – and not fulfilling ourselves – again, who knows what that is.

There is nothing wrong with reaching our self-described potential, so long as it is our ideal, and not society's or someone else's ideal. When we are working on our own ideas, living our own life on our terms, we are less stressed out, experience less anxiety and fear as a result. Why? Because the more in control of our lives we are, the less stress fear and anxiety we experience. Control is the key word here. When we feel things are out of control we get more stressful, fearful and worried.

When we are in control of our lives, we feel more confident, positive and ready to try new things, without stress or fear and anxiety.

However, when we are motivated by another's or even society's idea of who we should be we can become fearful, experience much more anxiety (restlessness) and yes, experience more stress.

Why? Because there is a lack of control, and it's not our true desire to live, as others would have us. Human beings are at their best when they are independent of these things.

Think about it, how you feel when someone or something is making you do what you don't want to do. That's right, you get worked up, frustrated, angry, all of which means you are experiencing more stress, anxiety, and fear.

They say that no two people are exactly alike and I believe that. However, in this way, we are all the same, as from the time we are small, we are told what to do and say so, and we live our lives in the expectations and shadow of someone else's wants, needs, and desires. It's the primary reason we aren't satisfied because we really haven't learned to just be ourselves and enjoy just being that, and do what we want, which is basically to take control of our lives.

Let's look at a practical application of that. I'm going to use a point of dissatisfaction many people have and that's with their vocation or job as an example.

How many of you work in a job that you really, I mean really hate? Yet every day you get up, get dressed, and drive to work – in slow or stuck traffic –to that job you just hate. Working eight, maybe longer hours, with people you don't like, dealing with the office politics and all, and you just hate it, you hate it to death. However, you do it, day in and day out. So why just not go? Why not just say to yourself, "I know I have responsibilities, but I simply can't do this anymore!

But then it's about here that your fear and anxiety kick in, "That would be irresponsible; I have bills to pay and mouths to feed!" All which are valid concerns, but again are you in control or not?

Because generally in this situation you are not in control, you will definitely feel more stress along with stress and anxiety because you feel "trapped" by your circumstances.

While that idea of responsibility, making a living, and providing are noble in themselves, sooner or later, we have to ask ourselves, "Am I happy?" Now you've no doubt heard that happiness is a choice and that is true but is it happiness is based on YOUR choice, or someone else's.

I worked for nearly 40 years and yet and I have to admit I really wasn't happy doing what I did to earn a living. I always felt I was missing something. The fact is that I hated getting up and going to work, which was usually in a job I didn't like, working with people I didn't really want to hang around socially.

Don't get me wrong, I was married during most of that time and I loved my wife, and wouldn't trade a minute of being with her. I also needed the insurance to cover her medical needs, and I was grateful for that. However, even she knew I wanted to be something else, specifically a writer and speaker. She would tell me to quit and try that, but again, those responsibilities weighed heavy.

I wanted to be a writer from my youth. I always was creating and writing stories, and I loved teaching. Yet from early in my adult life the expectations of my parents, specifically my dad, and an ill-advised teen relationship changed that. My girlfriend at the time became pregnant and the only option I could see was that we get married. Of course, there was significant pressure from our families to bring the child into the word with married parents (this was the 70s). I loved my daughter, and even my wife, still at the time I wasn't in control. I joined the Army where I stayed for 13 years.

CHAPTER 1-WHAT DRIVES US

My dreams of being a writer faded into the dust. As life would have it, that marriage failed and I lost custody of my daughter, and I began my career in the Army.

Later during an assignment to Korea, I would meet my second wife; we were married and remained married so for 30 years, until her death in 2013.

Therefore, even after leaving the Army I worked a regular job to support us, pay the bills, etc.

However, after leaving the Army faced with what to do in my life, my writing dream came alive again and I began to write, howbeit on the side.

As I said, right after that heart attack in 2000, and

learning about stress to help me cope, I wrote a book on how 911 Dispatchers could cope with stress, then created a seminar for it and taught it to 911 Dispatchers across the US.

Only at the time, it didn't provide enough income to provide a good enough living for my wife and me, especially with all her medical bills. Moreover, I couldn't devote the attention that it takes to be a full-time writer.

So I was still a bit frustrated, but I did understand that this was the way things had to be at the time, and I learned to balance (a very important word to remember), my wants, needs with those of another.

CHAPTER 1-WHAT DRIVES US

Yet the key thing about this was that for at least partially I was in control of what I wanted to do. I learned that there is a difference between I have to do and I want to do. That difference is "choice". I learned I could limit the frustration by realizing that I chose to do whatever it took to support us and that in effect was a bit of control.

Now saying that I didn't choose our cancers or watching the horrible outcome of her cancer, and I know she didn't either. However, as I will tell you, later on, that is life, and I also learned that while we can't control the things that happen to us, we could control how we will react to them.

Additionally, we have more control of our lives than

we might believe.

After she died, faced now with my future, but in shock and grief about losing her (all normal emotions), I made some bad choices. You can read about this in my book, "My Waffles are Cold – A Man's Guide to Abusive Women."

Yet after that incredibly stressful experience, I again found that no matter what happens in life, even bad choices can be turned around for good.

Therefore, I decided that in life for whatever time that might be, I would follow my dream. I decided that I was going to do what I had dreamed of my whole life. I've since remarried to a woman that believes in my dream and affords me the time and support I need to do it.

I also have a comfort knowing my deceased wife is happy as she looks at me from above.

Again, control is the operative word. In scientific studies about stress, it's been long known that the less control you have the more stressed you will become. Now when I say, "Stressed", it will be important to remember that stress is of two types, "Negative" and "Positive".

I will define those two types in Chapter Three but remember now that when we talk about reducing stress we are talking about the negative sort.

CHAPTER 1-WHAT DRIVES US

Now, I realize that some people are actually happy in their chosen profession, but that is because it's chosen by them and they believe it's their calling.

There is nothing wrong with enjoying what you do, so long as it's YOUR calling and choice and not what someone else wants you to do. Again, it's really about control, specifically who's controlling your life?

For the most part the people I've met I have met many people in my life, who will answer that they are not in control, and there is nothing more fearful, and causes more anxiety than not having control of one's life; even if everyone else thinks it's noble to lay our control aside to do something we don't enjoy. All they feel is restless all the time and ask themselves what life is all about?

Again, ask your friends about how much they enjoy their job, or their vocation. You will likely hear them say, "I just feel like I should be doing something else."

How many times have you seen a movie about a man or woman working at a job they hate? They have responsibilities to be sure but every day they're stressed out and hating the point of even getting up in the morning.

Then one day they get up, pack up their desk, and walk out the door! They don't seem to care about the consequences; they just know they can't do that job one more day!

You looked at them and said, "Yeah I wish!" Again, that person decided one day that their freedom from fear and bondage to that fear had a breaking point. They knew if they didn't go that moment, they might be forever shackled to that desk. That might have been succeeding at that job, you know, reaching their potential!

Then they saw that they weren't working for anything but someone else's idea of potential, not their own. I can tell you that day they felt fear, but not of losing their job, but of being deluded enough to think they would reach their potential that way.

If they were ever going to reach their own full potential, they know wouldn't be there, at that desk, working for this or that company. How they would provide, or take care of their debts wasn't the issue. They had heard that if you do something that you really love doing the money would be there.

Therefore, off they went, and for the people I know who did it, it worked out just fine. Yet you say, "But I hate my job, but I just can't do that!"

Fine, a more practical way is to follow my dad's advice, "A wise person looks for his dream (true vocation) by preparing for it before leaving their job."

In other words, to get to where you want to, you must prepare for it. For myself, it took a while to get to do what I'm doing now. As I said, I couldn't be a full-time writer before, and it frustrated me. Yet knowing that the circumstances – even though they were not my choice – nevertheless, I chose to accept them for what they were, and I did what I could on the side – in my time – in order to prepare for that day when I could do what I really wanted to do.

What that did was to make me feel like a writer and more in control of my life. So while you might not be able to completely follow your dreams and goals now, there are things you can do in the interim to give you the feeling of control until you are able to "pull the switch" completely.

There is always more flexibility when we are in control, but there is no flexibility when someone else is in control, and we allow them or even circumstances to control our destiny. The more flexibility and control we have the less stress fear, and anxiety we experience.

That's a key point whenever we talk about coping with stress, fear, and anxiety. Why? Because those who are doing what they love are happier, more fulfilled, and less stressed, and have less fear and anxiety as a result.

CHAPTER ONE EXERCISE

Question 1: Do you feel in control of your life

most of the time? If not, in what areas, i.e.; job,

family, etc.

_____

_____

_____

_____

Question 2: What could you do to get more control

in the areas where you lack it?

_____

_____

_____

_____

CHAPTER 1-WHAT DRIVES US

_____

_____

_____

_____

_____

_____

CHAPTER 2 THE DIFFERENCE

BETWEEN FEAR & ANXIETY

As I said before, we will look at the definition of stress in the next chapter. For while they are linked together with stress, in that they determine the stress response we will have to a given situation, fear and anxiety are two different emotions and need to be individually defined.

One thing true of us all is that have all experienced fear and anxiety at one point or another in our lives.

In fact, we might even be experiencing them now while reading this book, thinking of something that is either right in front of you, or that we think may happen in the future. Perhaps some bad news you just received, or even anxiety about life in general at this point in your life.

However, we have to understand that as long as we are alive, we will have fear and anxiety, the goal is not a total elimination of these, but to lessen them to the extent possible.

Both are emotions just like any emotions such as sadness or happiness, or anger. Emotions can be a blessing or a curse, it's all about whether they help us or harm us. For instance, sadness can help us genuinely grieve a loss, but it can also indicate depression. It all depends on the circumstances.

CHAPTER 2 THE DIFFERENCE BETWEEN FEAR & ANXIETY

As any emotion, fear and anxiety come from our thinking, or the thoughts we have cause us to feel the way we feel.

When we think a fearful or anxious thought, we experience those emotions that correlate to that thinking. For an example, if you go to a scary movie, and watch all the scary things that are happening on the screen you will most likely experience fear and anxiety.

Perhaps you don't like scary movies because you don't like the having those emotions. Yet nothing is really happening except that you are watching a scary movie on a screen, TV, with actors and props. It's just lights, makeup, eerie music and things jumping out of nowhere, which are all scripted and no one is really getting hurt. However, we could experience fear simply because of what is going on in our mind while watching it.

REAL FEAR VS. IMAGINED FEAR

Fear is a different emotion than anxiety because fear is based on a **real threat**, something we can see or sense and know that it's real.

A real circumstance such as getting robbed by a thief would cause fear because we can see the thief. He's not some actor, but a real person who is threatening to do us real harm.

It might be someone breaking into our house

because we can hear the door crash in, a window smashed. We're not thinking it up in our imagination, and that's the key difference between fear and anxiety.

Anxiety, or what I call fear's "evil twin, is all about our imagination. It's all about what we THINK is going to happen tomorrow, or even today, or even yesterday. In other words, it's subjective and not based on facts. Such as being in the scary movie. What makes us fearful during the movie is the thoughts we are thinking in our mind that actually put us in the scene. Therefore, when the monster, ghost, whatever is chasing the characters into the barn, we're – in our mind – right there with them.

Which is why we think, and sometimes shout out, "Don't go in there!" "Run that way!"

Now that's all good fun, and for the record, I love a good horror movie, but if we translate that "fear" into the real world, we have problems.

For instance, let's say you have to walk down a dark street at night on the way home. There you are, out there alone, and while you're walking, it seems every shadow is a thief, and every corner is full of disaster.

The longer you walk the harder it becomes to keep your mind from thinking of really bad things that could happen to you.

However, the fact is that there is nothing real out

there, but your mind can create some scenario where there is a danger, and suddenly you hear a noise and you start running like the wind. What was it? A cat, or a rat, or maybe the wind, you don't know, and you don't care. Your mind created the picture of something that wasn't there and told your body "RUN!" and so you did.

HOW DO THEY WORK TOGETHER

Fear and anxiety can work together to drive you crazy. As an example, where this could happen is a situation I know we've all could identify with. That is misplacing your wallet. We've all done that I'm sure that at one time or another. So what usually happens? Well, we calmly look for it while whistling a tune. Well not if you're like me, and the vast majority of humans on earth.

No, you more than likely jump up and down, check your online banking, yell at everyone at home to "FREEZE" (as if they stole it), and generally get yourself all worked up.

Why? Because you are thinking "Oh my God, my money, my cards, my license, they're gone!"

Here again is where we can see the difference between fear and anxiety. First, we have the immediate threat (fear), "My wallet's gone!" followed by the secondary fantasy (anxiety) thoughts about what someone might do with your money if they find your wallet. First, you notice the wallet's gone. Your mind thinks, "Oh no it's gone!" which is real, it's not a fantasy.

But then comes the anxiety, or if you will, "Fear based on Fantasy", which causes your mind to begin telling you all the bad things the "thief" will do with your cash, credit cards, ID, etc.

Usually, it's just about the time when your heart is about to give out from fear and anxiety that someone shouts out, "Here it is!" You calm yourself, say "thank God", and go about your business.

You might even be embarrassed that you made such a fuss. Isn't it funny that most times, you lose something you always find it – or someone else does - just when you're just about to lose your mind in fear and anxiety? We all do this from time to time, and we do it with different things that happen to us.

How about losing your car keys, you know, just before you're about to leave for work. Again, the connection between your thoughts and feelings (fear and anxiety) are on display.

For example, you look for your keys, look at your watch, look for your keys, and look again at your watch. Suddenly you notice that five minutes you gave yourself for the 20-minute drive to work isn't working out and you go into a panic.

Of course, your mind helps you out at this point.

Your anxiety spikes and you think, *"Oh no I'm going to be late…!" "Then when I get to work late the boss will fire me…I will be broke, lose everything – even the car… and die penniless on the streets!"*

This is all happening within a split second of discovering you can't find your keys, and already you're homeless and dying on the streets. Just five minutes before you were enjoying your morning, drinking your coffee.

What happened to your peace? FEAR, ANXIETY that's what. The fear generated by fearful thinking.

First the fear, (Oh no the keys are gone!), and then the anxiety (What you think will happen since you won't find them and will be late for work).

Again, we all do this and with a thousand things that happen to us all throughout the day. Most things that are imaginary and drive our anxiety haven't happened and most likely won't happen. However, our minds don't care, because "It knows, it knows THIS is going to happen!" I'm convinced our minds can be our worst enemy in these situations.

Don't believe me; just ask your mind anytime of the day what input it has for the day or the future. Trust me, just ask it, and see that results you get. Normally they'll always be less than encouraging. I've always had the feeling that after I die my mind thinks it will go on.

Have you ever looked on Google for medical information about some sickness you may be experiencing at the moment, or some mark or bump you found on your body?

Most people do that and find that instead of having a cold their mind will tell them it's Pneumonia. It's not a bump on your leg, its bone cancer, etc. Notice it's always the worst case scenario <u>IN YOUR MIND</u>.

The positive thinking mania that many are writing and speaking about is sweeping our world today, it's all good, and I will tell you it can help. However, how many times do you remember that positive meme when the heat is on?

Yeah, positive sayings and thinking can help, but in order to enjoy the cure, you also have to understand the disease. Which is that basically, that many of us are bent towards the negative with everything in our life.

As I said in the last chapter, using only the example of our jobs, but it's true of most other things as well. We don't feel in control of our life and so when we have something happen, such as losing a wallet or seeing a bump on our body, we immediately take the negative approach.

That's really the fuel of negative thinking, the perception of a lack of control. When things feel out of control, we get agitated and try to reestablish control. When we're exhausted and feel too many things are out of our control we become fatalistic and negative, pessimistic if you will about life.

Because many of us have lived a life where we didn't have control, it can seem we've learned to be negative. You might say it's almost hardwired into our being, and also because our world has become so negative as well as if we needed more help.

It's true we are products of our environment. This is even truer if we were raised by negative parents or other significant influences in our early life who passed it along to us. Again, this is why all the

positive thinkers are so successful in trying to get

people to think positively, but again, it takes more

than speeches and memes to change this in us, again

we have to understand the core reason – a

perception of a lack of control.

CAN FEAR BE GOOD?

What makes fear really different that anxiety is that

fear can be good while anxiety is usually bad. We've

seen that in the examples I've given here.

Remember the case of being robbed or someone

breaking into our house that motivated us to

ACTION that was necessary to protect ourselves

and defend our family. Therefore, in that case, fear is good.

On the other hand, anxiety is always about imagining something that might happen, such as the fantasy thinking after losing the wallet and is something we have to try to avoid.

Therefore, you can see that while fear and anxiety are different, they do intermingle a bit. We'll look at this more as we go on. For now, let's look at stress.

CHAPTER TWO EXERCISE

Question 1: Describe a situation where your mind went farther than the situation that was actually happening.

_____

_____

_____

_____

_____

_____

_____

Question 2: What do you think is the most

important thing to do immediately after getting

"surprised" by something you didn't expect?

_____

_____

_____

_____

_____

_____

_____

_____

_____

_____

_____

CHAPTER 3 - DEFINING STRESS AND

THE STRESS RESPONSE

Simply defined stress is pressure. We refer to the

daily pressures on us as "stressors". Stress is actually

a structural term that refers to the pressures placed

on physical structures such as gravity, weather, etc.

To give a small example, think of a pencil. Now if

you wanted to break that pencil in half you would

grab it with both hands and snap it in half. If you

notice when most people do this they place their

thumbs in the middle on either side to make it easier.

What happens though is that the pencil breaks right

CHAPTER 3 - DEFINING STRESS AND THE STRESS RESPONSE

---

at the point of the greatest pressure, which also happens to be at the pencil's weakest point. Have you noticed that the smaller the pencil gets the harder it is to break it? That's because the smaller it gets the more resistance against the pressure it has.

Notice also that the pencil breaks because of outside pressure (your hands), not of itself.

However, just like the pencil we usually break at our weakest point, especially when the outside forces are at work. We may be able to withstand that pressure for a while, but if it's continuous, we will sooner or later break from it, UNLESS we find a way to cope with the pressure.

Now in our lives, pressure is everywhere. From the weather to our work, health, responsibilities, pressure is all around us. How we respond to that pressure (stress) is directly related how we think (thoughts) about what is happening to us.

The pressure is never going away so long as we are alive.

However, while the stress is usually on the outside, we only sense it from the inside, and that is by our thinking. Remember: *"It's not what's without, but what is within!"*

TWO SOURCES OF STRESS

There are two sources of stress or pressure, which reside under two main categories: External and Internal.

These categories describe the stress we face in life.

EXTERNAL	INTERNAL
Daily Hassle and /Frustrations	Our individual beliefs and values
Threats to well-being	Individual coping mechanisms
Conflict	Individual perceptions of incidents
Family and Relationships	Faulty thinking, scary thoughts
Work and School	Negative Self-Concept

Factors that determine how we respond to stressful events. Individual, Vulnerability.

INDIVIDUAL DIFFERENCES

Whether a demand is external or internal it is still a

demand on us to cope, adapt, and adjust. However,

while most of life's events are not unique, as the

same things happen to all of us, our individual

response to each event can and often is unique to

each of us.

This means that the response to an event could

produce sadness or anger in one person, but it could

also produce happiness in another person. It all

depends **on the way an individual looks at it**.

Some people are going to view some situations as

more threatening than others, in the same way, that

others are going to be less reactive to pressure

situations than those who are more reactive.

These can be factors such as:

Individual Personality Traits

Individual Skills

Our Aptitude (ability to learn)

Our Motivation (what we desire to do)

Our Overall Life Experiences

Our Individual Coping Strategies

VULNERABILITY FACTORS

In addition, how a person reacts to an event and that

person's ability to cope with stress is further affected

by certain **vulnerability factors** such as:

Genetic Predisposition – Biological Traits passed

from parents.

Learned coping skills - Coping skills learned from

parents, peers.

Individual lifestyle – Other strains we place on

ourselves by our lifestyles such as

tobacco/alcohol/drug abuse or inactivity.

POSITIVE AND NEGATIVE STRESS

Stress isn't always negative. It can be positive too.

The difference between the positive (Eustress) and

negative (Distress) stress isn't so much the event but

how each event affects us, and again whether we

want it to happen (control).

As far as control, remember for now that we can't control the stuff on the outside. We can only control how we are going to respond to it.

Therefore, it's not in the "cause" but the "effect" that we are concerned with when we look at stress.

Distress is an appropriate word because negative stress can cause distress to our bodies and minds. When we talk about reducing stress, it is the negative stress that we want to limit or eliminate in our lives.

Positive stress is what happens when we are doing what we want, such as getting married, having a baby, attending the graduation of our children.

Again, it's about control because it's something we want to do.

Negative stress is called that because it's always something we don't want to do or to happen us and feel a lack of control. Negative stress fights against our will, so we fight back, and so we spend more energy (negative energy) on it. However, the reason we fight against it is because we feel a lack of control, and wishing it wouldn't be happening to us, we react negatively to it.

Irrespective of what is happening, because all kinds of things happen all the time, even if the event isn't something, we've planned or expected the way we react to it – negatively or positively – determines whether it's negative or positive stress.

THE BIOLOGY OF STRESS

As we saw stress is the result of pressure, and as we are biological beings, it is a biological function and its origins go way back in our DNA to the dawn of time. It has a design to enable us to adapt to and cope with our environmental changes.

For instance, let's say one of your ancestors was out hunting one day for food, say a rabbit, but instead ran into a bear. Now at the time, no one knows just how to cook a bear, so he could either run away or

risk getting eaten.

Therefore, the bear surprises your ancestor, and his

body has a couple of responses the first is a

cognitive awareness of a real threat - the bear. You

might know this also as the "Fight or Flight"

response. The bear is huge and so the man

experiences fear because the bear is right there in

front of him. He's seen what a bear can do to a man

that only fuels his fear. It is based on a REAL

threat, not something he imagines. He's not anxious

he's in fear.

The response of fear follows his thought to FIGHT

the bear or RUN back to the safety of the cave.
Because he has such a small spear and the bear is so
huge; he falls to plan two and runs from the bear.

Now, this is a split-second decision and based on his
need for survival. So choosing to "flight" his body,
in turn, has a response to the pressure that bear's
presence brought. His bodily response from the
stress response enables him to run (quickly) away
from the bear.

THE THEORY OF THE GENERAL

ADAPTATION SYNDROME

Earlier in the last century a man, a Dr. Hans Seyle

formulated this into a theory called The General Adaptation Syndrome", or GAS, (I always like that acronym for obvious reasons). This GAS goes into effect every time we experience a stressor – which is whatever is happening – and ensures your body can adapt to it. However, something to note. This response to a threat happens whether it's real or imagined, because of the mechanics involved.

When your mind perceives a threat, the body will automatically respond because the brain centers that handle fear trigger certain biological responses.

In my opinion, Dr. Seyle's greatest contribution, however, was to identify how stress negative stress, affected the body. He discovered in his research theory that in most cases sustained stress, that which occurs over a long time could lead to chronic diseases, such as cancer, heart disease, and other illnesses. He referred to them as "diseases of adaptation".

What he found is that negative stress primarily that which comes from anxiety, can wear the body down to the point that the immune system is compromised. That means that your body can have trouble fighting everything from the common cold to cancer and heart disease. In fact, about 75% of doctor visits are stress-related disorders or psychosomatic in nature.

That's why you might wonder why the waiting room and even emergency room is so crowded when you visit.

Now back to the man and the bear. The General Adaptation Syndrome goes into effect to help the man escape the bear.

The GAS consists of three stages, The Alarm Stage, the Resistance Stage and the Exhaustion Stage. Below is a brief breakdown of each.

STAGE ONE – THE ALARM STAGE

The Alarm Stage goes to work immediately upon the

entry of the stressor as it prepares the body for

defensive action. Some of the responses of the

Alarm Stage are:

Respiration Increases

Heart rate increases

Blood pressure increases

Muscles tense

Digestion is slowed

Sugar is released from the liver

Adrenaline is secreted

Blood gets thicker

Immune System is Suppressed.

In an emergency, any detection of a threat, a part of the brain called the hypothalamus commands the release of hormones (chemical messengers that control various body activities) from different places in the body.

The main stress hormones are epinephrine and norepinephrine. Epinephrine is produced by the adrenal glands, located just above the kidneys; norepinephrine is produced in many places.

Together, they stimulate a range of physical

responses in the body's organs. The heart rate speeds up, blood pressure rises, breathing grows deeper and faster, blood flow is rerouted from digestion to muscles, and blood clots faster.

Simultaneously, hormones release stored fats and sugars to provide a surge of energy. So that the man has near super strength to escape the bear.

If you ever heard of stories about people lifting a care off of someone who was trapped and wondered "Where did they get that strength?" Thank the Alert Stage for this.

STAGE TWO - THE RESISTANCE STAGE

During the Resistance Stage, the body attempts to return to a state of balance, or "homeostasis", once the threat is gone, and heart rate and other bodily functions decrease to normal levels.

What happens is the hypothalamus sends a hormone signal to a nearby gland called the pituitary. The pituitary gland then releases adrenocorticotropic hormone, also called ACTH. ACTH travels to the cortex (outer layer) of the adrenal glands.

The adrenal cortex responds by releasing hormones called glucocorticoids. These hormones keep blood sugar high to provide extra energy, just in case there is still the chance of further threats.

Therefore, the body remains in a state of semi-alert

as begins to calm down and return to normal.

STAGE THREE - THE EXHAUSTION STAGE

In the Exhaustion Stage, all resistance has ceased.

The body becomes depleted of its hormonal

reserves. The usual result of this is burnout.

While we all may have varied levels of resistance,

sooner or later we're going to get exhausted if the

stress isn't removed. Remember, like the pencil,

everyone has a breaking point.

Long term stress such as with those who experience

abusive relationships, combat conditions or high-stress jobs, can experience this stage. What happens is that there is a constant back and forth between the Alert Stage and the Resistance Stage until the body can no longer respond and return to "normal". Additionally, this is the crux of Post-Traumatic Stress Disorder (PTSD).

The important thing to remember is that you don't need a bear for the stress response to occur; remember it occurs every time you sense a threat whether real or imagined.

For instance, you could be sitting there reading a book (like this one), when suddenly you wonder if you mailed that important letter, or paid that credit

---

card bill. You can't immediately remember if you did and suddenly the Alert Stage begins, your heart begins to race, and all the other GAS responses begin to occur and the fact is that unless you verify whether you mailed it or not, paid it or not, you don't know.

Has a friend ever snuck up on you and said, "Boo!" and you were started! If yes, that startled feeling you experienced is the stress response, and it produced (fear/fight or flight) and it scared you. Just as a reminder, if that has happened, remember how you were scared and then angry when you heard your "friend" smile and say, "Got you!" I'll bet you felt like getting them, let's hope you didn't. However, remember, fear/anger. Just keep that link in mind.

There are a whole lot of things like this and other things – stressors - that happen all throughout the day. Sometimes they are real, and most times, they are imaginary. Remember how when we looked at fear and anxiety that it's apparent that you don't have to ever leave your bed in the morning for anxiety to appear. Your mind can "awake" with you and it can just start "thinking". If it's negative thoughts, you'll be experiencing anxiety before you throw the covers back. (In fact, you might just throw them back up over your head!) We are going to explore this in depth in coming chapters.

One of the issues with anxiety is that if it becomes chronic it can lead to psychological issues such as Post Traumatic Stress Disorder (PTSD) or Generalized Anxiety Disorder (GAD). We'll define GAD a little more in the next chapter.

If you have constant anxiety after a while, everything is a crisis; your mind never shuts off. Do you have insomnia? Well sometimes insomnia is a result of physical issues but many times, it's because your mind just ruminates all night about this issue and that problem. It just won't go to sleep.

I'll leave a total treatment of PTSD for another

book, as it's a more complicated subject. However, for now, understand that both PTSD and GAD can be the result of the stress response getting "stuck "as you fluctuate between the Alert and Resistance stages so that after a time you are always in some portion of fight or flight.

Just remember that the stress response is a biological (physical) as well as a mental issue. The stress response comes from your brain – thus your thinking. However, just like anything, it can get out of whack and when it does we have problems.

A stuck response can also lead to other issues as well. Remember how Dr. Seyle noted this was where the body – in the Exhaustion Stage - can break down, lessening its ability to fight disease?

This is because one important feature of your body's natural defense to disease and sickness is the immune system. If you go back to the responses of the GAS, you'll see that the immune system is suppressed. The reason for this is that the body needs all available resources to respond to the threat.

If the stress is chronic, then the hit on the immune system and so the body is incredible. That is the main reason why I believe my body began to break down, first with my heart attack and then with cancer. You can only take so much. No one is invisible.

Therefore, stress isn't anything to play with, and later we'll look at coping with it effectively.

CHAPTER THREE EXERCISE

Question 1: Name some negative stress that you have experienced in your life.

_____

_____

_____

_____

_____

Question 2: Name some positive stress in your life.

(Remember, the things that bring you joy and that you want to do.)

_____

_____

_____

_____

_____

_____

CHAPTER 4 – FEAR, ANXIETY & STRESS

Fear and anxiety like stress, are also biological in nature. In fact, when we experience those emotions our bodies go through the same biological processes in which the whole of our being are involved, physically and emotionally, and produce the responses of the GAS.

However, remember, that whether the threat is real or imagined, your body goes through the same processes. If your mind thinks it true, then as far as your body is concerned it is true.

The difference is in what kind of thoughts we have at the time and that will determine the emotional response.

The difference is that why you can't control a real threat, you can work to control the negative thinking that leads to anxiety and so help to eliminate those negative thoughts.

Let's look at a definition of fear, and then anxiety by Wikipedia.

"Fear is a feeling induced by perceived danger or threat that occurs in certain types of organisms, which causes a change in metabolic and organ functions and ultimately a change in behavior, such as fleeing, hiding, or freezing from perceived traumatic events. Fear in human beings may occur in response to a specific stimulus occurring in the present, or in

anticipation or expectation of a future threat perceived as a risk to body or life. The fear response arises from the perception of danger leading to confrontation with or escapes from/avoiding the threat (also known as the fight-or-flight response), which in extreme cases of fear (horror and terror) can be a freeze response or paralysis.

In humans and animals, fear is modulated by the process of cognition and learning. Thus, fear is judged as rational or appropriate and irrational or inappropriate. An irrational fear is called a phobia.

Psychologists such as John B. Watson, Robert Plutchik, and Paul Ekman have suggested that there is only a small set of basic or innate emotions and that fear is one of them. This hypothesized set includes such emotions as acute stress reaction, anger, angst, anxiety, fright, horror, joy, panic, and sadness. Fear is closely related to, but should be distinguished from, the emotion anxiety, which occurs as the result of threats that are perceived to be uncontrollable or unavoidable. The fear response serves survival by generating appropriate behavioral responses, so it has been preserved throughout evolution."

Source: Fear - https://en.wikipedia.org

So we see that humans, just like animals, respond to threats in order to protect ourselves, and fear of safety is the driving force.

Now, let's look at anxiety.

"Anxiety is an emotion characterized by an unpleasant state of inner turmoil, often accompanied by nervous behavior, such

---

as pacing back and forth, somatic complaints, and rumination. It is the subjectively unpleasant feelings of dread over anticipated events, such as the feeling of imminent death. Anxiety is not the same as fear, which is a response to a real or perceived immediate threat, whereas anxiety is the expectation of future threat. Anxiety is a feeling of uneasiness and worry, usually generalized and unfocused as an overreaction to a situation that is only subjectively seen as menacing. It is often accompanied by muscular tension, restlessness, fatigue and problems in concentration. Anxiety can be appropriate, but when experienced regularly the individual may suffer from an anxiety disorder."

Source: Anxiety - https://en.wikipedia.org

Now let's see how each works with the stress

response. For instance our earlier example with someone who breaks into your house. Let's say that you are home with the family, in bed, about to go to sleep for the night and suddenly an intruder breaks in.

Of course, you would be a fearful event. You don't know who it is, but you heard the door being kicked in, or a window being shattered. Therefore, you grab something to confront the intruder, like a bat, golf club, or even your gun.

On the other hand, you may not do any of those things and run to the closet with your family and call 911 on your cell phone. However, in both cases, you will be detecting the threat and experiencing fear because your safety and security are being threatened. Your body, therefore, would go through the Fight or Flight response.

You might say, "Well yeah, but I would be angry too!"

Absolutely, but something you may not know is that while anger is an emotion like fear, it actually comes, as a secondary reaction to fear. However, let's look at what happens when fear and anxiety are intermixed.

For instance, if you have children, you've no doubt gone shopping with them, and especially if they're young, you make sure to tell them to stay close by.

Well, let's say one day little Johnny wanders away from you. When you notice he's gone your Alert Stage fires up and you begin to call his name, searching for him, and as time goes on your mind begins thinking of all things that could be happening. You begin to think, "Oh my God he's been abducted, kidnapped!"

This wouldn't be unusual at all especially in the light of all the terrible situations we read about happening in the news. However, remember, you really don't know right now. He could just be lost or hiding in the nearest clothes rack playing hide and seek.

But you frantically call his name, looking and as you do anxiety, fear, rise as your mind begins to create those scary scenarios, and are about to lose your mind with worry when suddenly there is an announcement over the store's PA system:

"Will the parent of Johnny please come to the customer service desk; your son is here to be picked up?"

Now a sense of relief floods over you as you hurry to the customer service desk. However, on the way there, that fear you were experiencing, even though you know that everything is OK now, turns into anger. So that by the time you arrive and pick up Johnny you're ready to "kill him", yelling at him, *"Just wait until I get you home!" "You scared me to death!"*

The same switch from fear to anger can happen with

the intruder in your house. While going downstairs to confront the intruder, you may be fearful but that will quickly turn into anger if you do meet with an intruder. You may only have a book in your hand, but what a mighty book it will be in your warrior's hands!

Again, we are made this way and that process of reaction to the threat, GAS processes will take place, just when they did when Johnny got lost.

IMPORTANT! GAS RESPONSES WILL HAPPEN WHETHER THE SITUATION IS REAL OR IMAGINED!

The process is natural, it's how we're built, but the results of the process might now always be good. What is the "intruder" is not a burglar, but only your older son coming in from a long night out with his friends, and being dark, you club him in the head?

However, when we are responding to our thoughts and emotions – without evidence – we can cause unintended consequences.

In all our examples, when the anxiety we experienced outweighed the result this is because of what is called, Catastrophic Thinking.

CATASTROPHIC THINKING

In the example of the lost wallet, car keys and even

losing your child in the store, your mind took over and began to "Catastrophize" what was happening into a larger incident in your mind than it was, "making a mountain out of a molehill."

If you want to see, your fear and anxiety levels rise quickly add catastrophic thinking to whatever is really going on. In fact, most anxiety disorders have this as a driving force.

I remember when I was young, back before I knew what I knew, and I was getting out of the Army after 13-years. I had been in the Army since of was 18 and it was all I knew. Suddenly one day I had really bad palpitations of the heart, trouble breathing, etc., and thought I was having a heart attack. The more I thought of it, I was convinced I was dying.

This was long before my actual heart attack nearly 12-years later, I was relatively young and in shape. However, it was beginning to keep me from getting sleep and functioning. One night while having one of these attacks, I called the hospital night nurse who immediately knew what it was and she told me to get a paper bag and slowly breathe into it. She told me this because she could hear me hyperventilating on the phone. I did what she told me and I began to feel better.

What I was doing though was thinking of all kinds of crazy scenarios now that I would be coming home, with no job and transitioning to civilian life no idea of how to find one. I was married to my wife at the time and she relied on me for support.

Now being concerned would have been normal, I'm only human. However, I let my mind go and come up with all these worst-case scenarios and so found out early in my life how debilitating Catastrophic Thinking can be. When we get to coping tools, I'll give you some tips on how to control them.

ANXIETY

As we've seen in the definition, and from what we've talked about so far, anxiety is based on ongoing worry, dread, that may or may not be based on specifics. We all get anxious from time to time.

Sometimes we can pin it down to something (worry about an upcoming test, or medical procedure), and other times not.

For example, you're worried about a test you are studying for because you think you might fail it, or you're an upcoming medical procedure, such as surgery, might go wrong.

In reality, you really don't know what's going to happen. If you studied for your test then you should pass it. If you're going to a competent surgeon, there should be a need to worry about the procedure.

The only truth at this point is the fact that you have

a test coming up, or that you have a medical procedure that is scheduled.

That would be it for now, but then the anxiety comes in to complicate it. Think how too much anxiety could get someone to cancel the test, or even cancel the surgery because the anxiety/worry over the results would be too great. It happens a lot. This is really simple fear about something that is real, but then anxiety about a result that hasn't happened yet.

How about another example. Let's say the boss tells you at 8 am that he/she wants to see you at 5 pm, or the end of the day.

You don't know what it was about, or what was going to happen, and so you are anxious about an upcoming event that you had no idea what the outcome will be.

Again, in the end, no matter what, you will likely find out it was nothing like you imagined, and going to his office at the end of work found out it was indeed there nothing to dread.

However, because of the anxiety, you experienced, about a result you couldn't actually know, you likely spent the whole day worrying about what was going to happen just to find out when the time came it was nothing at all.

As you can see, anxiety can absolutely ruin your day or even week if you don't put brakes on it.

GENERALIZED ANXIETY DISORDER (GAD)

Sometimes anxiety is "generalized", or there is no specific cause or reason. When this is persistent and interferes with living a productive life, psychologists call this, Generalized Anxiety Disorder or GAD. GAD is always based thinking that something bad is going to happen, some doom looms, even though you can't exactly explain why you feel that way, or there is no perceivable threat in view. In essence just an intense sense of worry or unease that can be debilitating.

GAD is generally the reason millions go to see mental health professionals about anxiety, insomnia, feeling 'stressed out'. It's not too difficult to treat but requires more than just a few visits. Many people rely on pharmaceuticals to get by, and again, I'm not a doctor or psychiatrist, and I wouldn't dare tell you not to take what you prescribed. However, think about it. To me, it's like putting a band aid on an open chest wound. It may cover the problem for a while, but at what cost in money, time and productivity? I know because I've been prescribed a medication or two over my lifetime. However, for me coming to grips with the mechanics of stress, anxiety and fear were enough to finally deal with the issue at its source and stop taking them. Keep reading to see what I discovered, and especially in the next chapter on Thoughts, Emotions, and Actions.

Again, over time anxiety, because it, like fear and stress is so linked to linked to our biological processes, that if it runs free it can begin to wear down our bodies and can lead to those diseases of adaptation that Dr. Seyle wrote about in his theory.

For instance, he wrote that one particular reason for this is the suppression of the immune system in the stress response.

When your immune system is suppressed, the body

simply cannot protect itself as it normally would. When the Alert Stage is sustained, or continually triggered, the immune system can become chronically compromised, leading to diseases of adaptation.

As I talked about in the beginning, I've had firsthand experience this process.

Remember how I wrote about how my wife had battled cancer for 14-years and died in 2013. As I said, prior to that, she had numerous battles with the ravages of the disease, and in October of 2009 received what would be her final diagnosis.

In that same month, I too was diagnosed with

cancer, and I remember my experience with teaching stress over the previous 10 years, and while using my tools I taught others helped me cope, helped me through it, I also know that my cancer likely happened because of the stress, anxiety, and fear I experienced as a caregiver.

I know this because most cancer is genetic, and I had no other incidences of that my type of cancer in the family.

Because I constantly feared AND had anxiety for my wife's safety and wellbeing, and even though I used all the stress coping tools that I knew, I could feel my body begin to break down.

This leads to a point to remember. That is even though you may know what is happening to you if it is a new event, something you never experienced before will require extra attention to cope with it.

For anyone who has been through this or is going through that experience of being a caretaker knows it's extremely stressful. Your mind is always filled with "what ifs", and whether or not this day or the next is their last.

Now with my diagnosis of cancer as well I had to deal with my own mortality and questions that brought, such as how to care for my wife – should I precede her, and whether or not I would get to see, my grandchildren grow up. I got so busy caring for her that I didn't have, or take the time for my own self-care.

However, as it happened, my wife died, and I survived.

Therefore, the physical effects of chronic stress are real. However, it doesn't just have to lead to a serious disease or sickness.

For instance, you have experienced some of that negative stress, fear or anxiety, I ask you how many colds or flue do you have a year? It's normal to catch a cold or the flu once in a while, but some people catch it several times a year.

Do you have arthritis? Did you know that certain

kinds of arthritis, specifically Rheumatoid, are due to a compromised immune system? Do you have heart disease? Cancer? While those diseases may not be always caused by stress, fear, and anxiety, but it's a strong possibility that you have been under the negative effects of stress for a considerable amount of time and because your natural immunity was compromised, and didn't help the situation.

There are also other negative contributing factors that can be nothing but destructive to your health. People who are chronically stressed are more likely to smoke cigarettes, or drink alcohol excessively and even use illegal substances, none of which is particularly good for your body.

ANXIETY = NEGATIVE THINKING!

Anxiety is more than anything else is negative thinking. Negative thinking leads to negative emotions such as anxiety, and chronic anxiety to lead to sickness and disease.

Therefore, it's important to find out just how many negative emotions you may be experiencing and more important how to deal with them. To begin that we need to look at the link between thoughts, emotions, and actions.

CHAPTER FOUR EXERCISE

Question 1: How much anxiety do you feel you

have on a daily basis?

_____

_____

_____

_____

Question 2: Can you give an example where you have faced a situation where you thought Catastrophically? If so, what have you learned to help you not do that in the future.

_____

_____

_____

_____

_____

_____

_____

_____

_____

_____

Question 3: Do you suffer from many colds, more than one flu a year? Are you frequently tired, worn out or restless? Do you think it's because you're chronically stressed?

_____

_____

_____

_____

CHAPTER 4 – FEAR, ANXIETY & STRESS

CHAPTER 5 – THOUGHTS, EMOTIONS,& ACTIONS

So far, we have learned a lot about stress, anxiety, and fear, and we learned that our emotions come from our thoughts, and how deadly and debilitating negative thoughts such as those that produce anxiety can be.

Now let's look at that thought/emotion/action connection more closely. This chapter will be longer than the rest, but it's important to learn this connection because it's to key to understanding how our thinking is the driving force behind negative stress, fear, and anxiety.

CHAPTER 5 – THOUGHTS, EMOTIONS,& ACTIONS

When we are dealing with the stresses of life, we may have the tendency to look on things that are happening to us negatively. As I said in Chapter 1, if we're honest it would seem that most of us are really just negative about everything that happens in our lives sometimes, nothing is ever enough.

Let's look at an example of that I'm sure that has happened to most of us.

Let's say you're driving somewhere and someone goes through a stop sign and nearly hits you. You yell out "look out!", and avoid a crash but afterward, you might say, "Wow that was close!", but then just as quickly you follow that with, "Oh my God, what if they would have hit me!" or even, "That nut almost killed me!"

You even may have had someone with you and might have said, "Well be thankful they didn't." However, just as fast you reply to their statement, or maybe think, "Yeah, but what if they had hit me?"

Notice how much you go back in forth in your mind in just a few seconds. Of course, we should be thankful that that driver didn't hit us and cause us an accident, but it seems sometimes we just can't let that go at that.

However, it seems that there just has to be that extra thought. I call them the "but's", or that little bit we just have to add to the context of what really happened. We do it so fast at times that we think it's just a normal response.

Going back to the car keys that we lost. Remember the fact that we lost the keys is the only thing that is really happening at that moment, but then our minds add all the scary scenarios that our minds think that will happen, again switching to the negative outcome. "I'm going to get fired!"

Even after we find the car keys, we're still pumped up a bit with the negative emotions; imagine then if finally going to work you hit a traffic jam? Then after you get to work, that's the day the boss wants to see you at 5 pm? Unless you grab your thoughts, you're going to be an anxious mess by the end of the day.

As I explained before, that just seems to be the way we're built. However, at what cost has taken the negative approach ever done us any good at all? How much better and less stressful if we took the adversities positively.

If we were to take it down a notch, and just look for the keys without adding negative imaginary symbolism to it, scaring ourselves, we would have a much nicer morning, and maybe find the car keys much faster.

This is true with most of what we react to during the day. All day long, we are bombarded by things –

stressors – that cause us to have to cope with, adjust to and react to them. Some of these stressors we have to make split-second reactions to, and others do not require us to react to not as quickly.

Yet in our mind, we get those two things mixed up, and react quickly to the stressors that could wait, and procrastinate about those things that need doing now.

This is because it can seem that everything is coming at us all at once and it can get hard to keep up at times.

However, unless we want to give up in life and throw in the towel, we have to learn to deal with stressors, in a positive and constructive way. So just how do we do that?

By separating fact from fiction. As we've seen, our minds can take us into the future and speed back to our past in a flash. We have to learn how to arrest these thoughts and put them in the proper perspective.

One way to do this is to write them down. To do this as a practice, take out a piece of paper and draw three columns. Now label the first column "Event", the second "Feelings", and the Third "Actions".

When you're done, it should look something like this.

EVENT	FEELINGS	ACTIONS

Good, now that you have that, let's use the near miss car accident as an example.

EVENT	FEELINGS	ACTIONS
Driver nearly hits you.	Fear, anxiety, anger.	Slam the breaks, honk your horn.

Now notice the mind/emotions link, which is fear and anger, and then the subsequent action in this chart. Remember anger follows fear. Just like in our example with the mom of little Johnny. First, she experienced.

First, you experienced fear and then once you determined you were all right, you experienced anger. However also notice at where the anger comes in. It comes with the anxiety. While the fear of almost getting hit is valid, your anxious thoughts, "He almost killed me!" caused that anger to act with even more aggression.

Just like that mom who lost her child in the store. First, you were anxious, fearful, then relieved, and then mad, yet the fear-fueled anxiety almost had you to act in anger towards Johnny even though he was all right.

The principle behind this is what Psychologists call The ABCs of Behavior, and it is the basis of the psychological theory of Cognitive Behavioral Therapy (CBT).

Most of what I've written in this book follows the model of CBT and what it simply means is what we think determines how we feel and that's how we act.

Let's break down CBT a little further.

"A" stands for the Actuating Event, or Events, such as losing your child or car keys or avoiding a near accident.

The Actuating Event could be anything at all that is happening to us; and here is the important part, whether it's real or imagined. Remember that "imagined" part because an actuating event doesn't have to be real to get us thinking about it and responding to it.

For instance, the Actuating Event with your boss telling you that they want to see you at the end of the work day. Remember how you might think of all kinds of scenarios that might happen, but none of which have HAPPENED YET, or may not happen at all.

All you know is that he/she wants to see you at the end of the work day. You let your mind go and it's going on overdrive, *"Omg, I was late, that's what it's about!"*

Then comes the end of the day and you at his office only to find out it was nothing. You would be relieved, but you even might be a little angry! Therefore, after you find out it was nothing you say,

"Boy boss, you scared me, I mean I sat in my office all day doing nothing but thinking about what you were going to do to me!"

Your boss could easily think, *"Well, they're a bit sensitive aren't they, wow, they had no productivity for the day because they thought I was going to yell at them."*

God forbid you to have an abusive boss who just found out you have yet another button they could push.

All this because once the anxious thoughts come in, there may be no end to what damage they could do. However, what happened during the day was that your body was in the Alert Response and it couldn't come down from it because (in your mind) the danger was still there.

So that by the time you arrived at the boss's office at 5 pm you were still in the "Fight or Flight" mode, even after finding out it was nothing. Subsequently, it may take a while to calm down (resistance stage), enough for you to reach homeostasis.

If this situation was prolonged, say in in high-stress environment, this may be a break the camel's back sort of situation, in which to "snap", and say or do something you might later regret.

Another example may be about sitting in a chair at home alone and suddenly you remember you forgot to pay your taxes, or pay a credit card bill.

Suddenly your body goes into the Alert Response, no differently than if a burglar just smashed through your window.

Remember if your mind thinks it, your emotions will

respond. If your body is constantly subjected to the Alert Stage with no significant adaptation (calming down), your response to stress will be on a greater level.

So what if after responding to the unpaid credit card you discover that you did pay it and because you didn't remember it, yet you responded to the threat in your mind anyway.

You see, emotions; fear and anxiety, anger, will respond to your thoughts. They can't differentiate between real or fantasy – only your mind/thinking can do that.

That's just how much powerful the mind it and why

it's critical to keep track of what we are thinking and separate fact from fiction, and keeping your mind from going to the negative. More on that in a minute.

I like to call these Actuating Events as "People, places and things", which pretty much covers whatever happens to us on a daily basis.

BELIEFS

The second part of the formula, "B", is our "Beliefs". This is a major part of the formula because we all have our different beliefs and views about how the world works, and the way things should be, and how people should act, do and say.

All this majorly effects how we are going to feel about a situation, and how we are going to think about an event.

What mainly determines our beliefs is our **EXPERIENCE** and our **MEMORY**. Experience being all the life experience we have had up to the present, to which we have committed to our memory, like a computer.

As we face an actuating event our minds begin to process it (as a computer would), and we begin to compare it against other experiences like it that we have stored in our memory.

We then assign the event a meaning and try to cope

and adjust to it.

Another part of how we form our beliefs that are formed over time throughout our life consist primarily of:

Underlying Assumptions/Beliefs/Judgments

Usually conditional conclusions we have about behavior and "how things should work" for us. The "should haves" and the "if only" live here.

Core Belief (schemas)

Our fundamental beliefs about others, the world, and ourselves. Our rules for "self-worth". For example, if we think, "If I make people happy, I'm OK. "If I don't make people happy I am a failure!"

That constitutes our rule for self-worth.

We can become pretty entrenched in our beliefs. They've been there a long time, but just because we believe them doesn't make them true, and that's important too.

Because there is a cost for our thoughts and emotions could be way out of line with what is really going on, and the cost is the Consequences, the "C" they can bring.

CONSEQUENCES

For an example, let's use the car near-miss car accident again to see where thoughts, beliefs lead to a consequence.

THINKING	BELIEFS	CONSEQUENCES
That crazy driver almost killed me!	They should follow the law, drive safely and pay attention.	Followed the guy five exits cutting in and out of traffic, while waving him the international sign for displeasure.

So this unattentive driver nearly hit's your car, that's a fact. It understandably frightens you, because your survival response (Alert Stage) kicked in. But you think, "He nearly killed me!" Of course, you don't know that, even if he did hit you.

Sure it would have been an accident, but how serious it would have been being something you don't know.

But the thoughts of that happening enrage your beliefs, your shoulds, and now you feel that he should pay! So with your sense of justice, you act on that belief, plus enabled by the adrenaline fueled stress response that is now causing you to "fight" instead of "fight".

So you believe so strongly in those beliefs, and because you're now mad at him, you drive like a maniac, trying to cut him off and throwing him the international sign for displeasure. However, in doing this not only did you violate your beliefs, you likely violated the law, while putting yourself, and him, in further danger (especially if he happens to have a gun, or stops and gets out of the car or a fight).

This is where most road rage occurs, and how many times have we read in the news where that went bad?

So are these beliefs about that driver valid? After all, you put a high regard on your life (who doesn't?) and believe all people should respect that. You also believe that all people who drive should obey the law and follow traffic devices and STOP! So far so good, I think those are pretty basic and reasonable beliefs.

However, while you believe that and it's valid, you have no idea why that driver was driving the way they were. After all, who hasn't done something quickly or even not been paying attention while driving?

Perhaps he too lost his car keys that morning and was hurrying to work, or maybe his wife (whom you didn't see or notice) was going into delivery and he was speeding to the hospital. What if that were so and so following him erratically you cause the accident you just missed, and you injure his pregnant wife?

You see you just don't know. Even if he was just being an aggressive driver, what do you hope to gain by driving as erratically as he drives?

All this because your beliefs, which are understandable and strong, were mixed with fear, then anger and because you allowed your thoughts free reign over the situation.

You have to catch yourself at the point of thought and don't allow the initial emotion to spiral into emotions that betray the truth of what you believe.

IRRATIONAL THOUGHTS

As we've seen, we may well have very understandable and valid beliefs and values, but we often find that our beliefs conflicting with reality. These are called Irrational Beliefs or thoughts. All of us have irrational beliefs. These beliefs are irrational not because they don't make sense or are not "noble", but because in reality, they are many times not reasonable or doable. Unfortunately, irrational beliefs can cause more stress and pressure on you as you strive to defend them.

Here are a few of them:

1. You must have love and approval nearly all the time from people who are important to you.

2. You must be completely competent in all your endeavors, or you must have real expertise or talent in something important.

3. Life must go the way you want it to. Things are

awful when you don't get your first choices.

4. Other people should treat everyone fairly. When people are unfair or unethical, they are horrible and rotten and are to be punished or avoided.

5. People and things should turn out better than they do turn out. It's awful and terrible when quick solutions to life's hassles are not forthcoming.

6. Your past is a strong influence on your behavior and must continue to affect you and determine your behavior.

7. You can find happiness by inertia, inactivity, or passivity.

Why are these thoughts irrational? After all, number

two sounds like a lofty goal to have. We all strive for perfection and believe we should be good at something. Yet just because an idea sounds rational, doesn't exactly make it so. When we bind ourselves to an irrational belief in an "all or none" stance, we are apt to be "kicked off our pedestal" when the conditions change – and they will.

For instance, when we believe that everybody must like us all the time, we will find it hard to accept or tolerate someone not liking us. Subsequently, we put pressure on ourselves to perform for them, and try to please them. Consequently, we get stressed when we perceive that they don't like us, or we feel their disapproval. This was the example and lesson we talked about in Chapter One.

You may not know this, but it is generally estimated that approximately 80% of the people you are going to meet in your lifetime are either not going to like you, or could care less about you, or just too busy with their own life. That only leaves a group of about 20% that you can possibly gain friends, confidants, and mentors.

If we insist that we want 100% approval from everyone we meet in life, we create an expectation that is unrealistic. It's is "setup" and a sure formula for feeling bad, rejected and useless.

COGNITIVE DISTORTIONS

Cognitive distortions are simply mistakes in thinking, and they are prime examples of negative thinking. Like Irrational Thoughts, they are based on the unrealistic expectations of others and ourselves.

See how many of these Irrational Thoughts that you can identify with.

1. Mind reading: You assume you know what people think without having sufficient evidence of their thoughts. "He thinks I'm a loser."

2. Fortune telling: You predict the future; things will get worse or there is danger ahead. "I'll fail that exam" and "I won't get the job."

3. Catastrophizing: You believe that what has

happened or will happen is so awful and unbearable that you won't be able to stand it. "It would be terrible if I failed."

4. Labeling: You assign global negative traits to yourself and others. "I'm undesirable" or "He's a rotten person."

5. Discounting positives: You claim that the positives you or others attain are trivial: "That's what wives are supposed to do, so it doesn't count when she's nice to me." "Those successes were easy, so they don't matter."

 6. **Negative filter**: You focus almost exclusively on the negatives and seldom notice the positives. "Look

at all the people who don't like me."

7. Overgeneralizing: You perceive a global pattern of negatives on the basis of a single incident. "This generally happens to me. I seem to fail at a lot of things."

8. Dichotomous thinking: You view events or people in all-or-nothing terms. "I get rejected by everyone" or "It was a waste of time."

9. Should Have's: You interpret events in terms of how things should be rather than simply focusing on what is. "I should do well. If I don't, then I'm a failure."

10. Personalizing: You assign a disproportionate

amount of blame to yourself for negative happenings and fail to see that certain events are also caused by others. "The marriage ended because I failed."

11. Blaming: You focus on the other person as the source of your negative feelings, and you refuse to take responsibility for changing yourself. "She's to blame for the way I feel now" or "My parents caused all my problems."

12. Unfair comparisons: You interpret events in terms of standards that are unrealistic; for example, you focus primarily on others who do better than you do and find yourself inferior by comparison. "She's more successful than I am" or "Others did better than I on the test."

13. Regret orientation: You focus on the idea that you could have done better in the past, rather than on what you can do better now. "I could have had a better job if I had tried" or "I shouldn't have said that."

14. What if?: You keep asking a series of questions about "what if" something happens, and fail to be satisfied with any of the answers. "Yeah, but what if I get anxious? Or what if I can't catch my breath?"

15. Emotional reasoning: You let your feelings guide your interpretation of reality; "I feel depressed, therefore my marriage is not working out."

16. Inability to disconfirm: You reject any evidence

or arguments that might contradict your negative thoughts. When you think, "I'm unlovable," you reject as irrelevant any evidence that people like you. Consequently, your thought cannot be refuted: "That's not the real issue. There are deeper problems. There are other factors."

17. Judgment Focus: You view yourself, others, and events in terms of evaluations of good bad or superior-inferior, rather than simply describing, accepting, or understanding. You are continually measuring yourself and others according to arbitrary standards, finding that you and others fall short. You are focused on the judgments of others as well as your own judgments of yourself. "I didn't perform well in college" or "If I take up tennis, I won't do well" or "Look how successful she is. I'm not successful."

Irrational Beliefs and Cognitive Distortions are usually at the root of our core beliefs, judgments that drive our emotions and so our actions. Therefore, because they are in fact negative thoughts, we will have negative emotions and actions.

AUTOMATIC THOUGHTS

Automatic Thoughts or "NAT"s are what the name implies. That is, they come into our minds automatically, they just "pop in" seemingly out of nowhere. We have a multitude of thoughts that come flooding into our minds all day long.

Sometimes just random, or "running thoughts", which appear to be disjointed, or somewhat together in meaning. Sometimes they come quickly, and all at once. If you've ever been overwhelmed with thoughts, you have the idea.

What can happen with so many random thoughts is if that if they are negative, they can trigger fear as your ability to keep up with them and that can become quickly overwhelming.

Our previous examples of the car keys, the lost child, the lost wallet or the near-miss accident, we looked at Catastrophic Thinking and saw that it does nothing except get us all worked up about nothing.

Irrational Beliefs, Cognitive Distortions, and Automatic Thoughts are usually to blame for Catastrophic Thinking. If we correct these errors in our thinking, we go a long way to counter Catastrophic Thinking.

Life isn't that absolute, as I've found in my experience. Every day we get up and have a choice, to take the positive approach to life, no matter what, or look at everything in a negative light. We can capture our thoughts, or let them roam free, and drive us crazy.

That's our choice. It's not easy to change the way we

think and believe, but nothing worthwhile is easy. However, it all begins with practice. You might have heard people say, "Practice makes perfect!" That makes a good internet meme or inspirational poster, but it's not true. Who is perfect? I don't care how much I practice anything I'll never be perfect at it.

Nobody is. Better to say, "Practice makes better." That's at least reasonable and obtainable. I've been playing and practicing the guitar for more than 50 years, and I'm pretty good, but I'm far from perfect. Besides, I have more fun if I just try to get better, and that's all life really is, just getting better.

CHAPTER FIVE EXERCISE

Question 1: What negative thoughts, irrational beliefs, or examples of catastrophic thinking have you experienced?

_____

_____

_____

_____

_____

Question 2: Where do you see areas to improve on? Can you see how these changes could reduce your stress, anxiety and fear?

_____

CHAPTER 5 – THOUGHTS, EMOTIONS,& ACTIONS

_____

_____

_____

_____

CHAPTER 6 – WHAT KIND OF PERSONALITY ARE YOU

When we look at stress, anxiety, and fear, we've seen we have to look at our entire being. The last chapter we looked at the connection between mind and emotions, Negative thinking, Irrational Beliefs and Cognitive Distortions and saw that they are at the root of how we think, feel and ultimately how we act.

Negative thinking is thought to be a product of our upbringing and environment. Again, if our parents were negative people, always seeing the mountain for the molehill chances are that we will too.

Social scientist says that our personalities are formed early in life and determine our approach to it. Therefore, we have learned that our behaviors as well from our parents or significant others as we grew, and then carried those characteristics, beliefs, and values into our adult lives.

If our parents exhibited high anxiety, we're likely to as well. Regardless of where it came from the important thing to remember is that stress, fear, and anxiety are all directly related as one launches the other.

If we lack appropriate coping skills to our daily stressors then we are more likely to be stressed out, anxious and fearful. If we didn't learn how from our parents or upbringing it's never too late to learn. To begin let's start with what type of personality we may possess.

Essentially, there are two personality types that we will look at, Type A and Type B. Of late, there has been a third category, Type C, but it's more a bit of the middle ground between A and B, so we'll keep it simple. Let's take a look at a chart of both and see which one fits your personality more. Pay particular note that they are categorized as "Healthy" and "Unhealthy" traits of each. Take a look on the next page to view the chart.

Are You Mostly Type A or Type B?

	Anger/ Confrontation	Ambition	Time	Taking Charge	Confidence	Approach to Change, New Things
Unhealthy A	Hostile, hot reactor	Driven, fiercely competitive	Ruled by the tyranny of time	Aggressive, domineering	Arrogant	Reckless
Healthy A	Easily Angered	Very ambitious	Feel urgency	Forceful	Self-promoting	Risk-taker
Healthy A	Slow to Anger	Dynamic, no need to prove yourself	Conscious of time, but not ruled by it.	High Energy and allowing	Radiance, confidence	Adventurous
Healthy B	Gentle, even-tempered	Calm, no need to prove yourself	Conscious of time but not ruled by it	Low-key and allowing	Quietly Confident	Inquisitive
Healthy B	Shy away from confrontation	Laid back	Lose trace of time easily	Hesitant	Unsure, hold back	Cautious
Unhealthy B	Fear Confrontation	Apathetic, lack drive	Oblivious to time	Passive	Low self esteem, fear taking a stand	Fear change

157

Now depending on where you find yourself you may be either Type A or Type B, healthy or unhealthy types of each or you might you may be a sort of mix between them (Type C).

This isn't set in stone, but it may help you see how you're "engineered" to react to stress, anxiety, and fear.

Years ago it was originally thought that Type A's were the type to have a myriad of medical issues such as heart attacks or strokes, but recent studies show that may not be the case with all Type As.

However, as we've seen with stress and its effects on the immune system there can be a significantly greater risk of these threats when stress levels are elevated. Of course, lifestyle, diet, whether or not there is exercise or not all play a factor as well.

I like to think of myself as a recovering unhealthy Type A, which means I'm still working on it.

I've mellowed with age along with the things that I've mentioned that have happened to me over the years. So I actually now pay particular attention to signs that show me I need to back off and slow down.

However, one thing that seems to be agreed upon, and is my experience, is that Type As, especially unhealthy types, have a lot more negative thinking traits and so more fear and anxiety.

When it comes to catastrophic thinking, Type As seem to have a lot more trouble with keeping thoughts in the NOW.

I believe a lot of that came from my parents, siblings and the general environment I grew up. Don't get me wrong my parents were good people and raised me correctly, but somehow I picked up on the angst of the time (the 60s and 70s) in American and the world. However, I remember many times little molehills grew into mountains rather quickly.

However, as I grew, it seemed to get worst and while

CHAPTER 6 – WHAT KIND OF PERSONALITY ARE YOU

I've always been what they call "high-strung", I got a lot worse as I got older.

As I said in the beginning, I feared almost everything, to the point of being afraid of my own shadow. If I got a letter from the IRS my mind immediately told me that I was going to prison! Of course, I would hide it away for weeks, until I couldn't stand the suspense any longer, only to find that was a refund check for a $1.95. Therefore, for a couple of days, I stressed myself out over nothing. That's changed a lot because I've learned the things about the kind of things that happened to me over the years that I've relayed to you so far.

The first thing I did to improve was to address my

Type A characteristics. For a while in my life EVERYTHING, had to happen RIGHT NOW, nothing, absolutely nothing could wait. But after a while of addressing the irrational thinking and cognitive distortions which Type A has a lot of, that too began to lessen, and I began to relax and deal with life as it was, one day at a time.

As I said my Type A was of the unhealthy type and so dialing that back wasn't easy, but I had to do it. Here is one of the little things that I did that you could do. It's very easy, takes a little practice, but really works.

At the beginning of the day write down, all the things that your mind says just have to be done that day. That's it, just that one day. You'll likely come up with a list of a few pages.

Now take that list and pare it down to just the things you can realistically do that day. Call each task "project". Again, you'll have a bit of difficulty at first, but what helped me was to have a watch or clock nearby. If you are a Type A you won't have problems with having enough clocks, you likely have them all over the house and office.

Now, write down the hour you're going to start the project, and then what you are going to need to do in that hour to get it done.

Once you get it done, move on to your next project.

CHAPTER 6 – WHAT KIND OF PERSONALITY ARE YOU

At the end of the day you'll find that with eating, driving to and from work, and all the other things that take up a day, you don't have a lot of time. At the end of the day, reflect on how many projects you actually got done. At first, you may be angry that you couldn't do them all, but again, ask yourself, how much can you really accomplish in the little time you actually have in one day?

One of the things you find is that time management isn't just a skill; it's a reality if you're going to get anything done in a day. However, the fact of the matter is that Type As are really not that good at time management, nor multitasking as they think they are.

The fact is that they can do a lot of different things at once, but they have difficulty completing one task before moving on the other.

So that at the end of the day they are angry and disturbed at themselves for what they couldn't do, and end up with problems like insomnia, chronic stress, anxiety and yes, fear.

The point of this exercise is that once you look at the things you want to do vs. what is realistic, you'll find yourself with only a few things that can be done in one day. However, THAT'S OK, it really is! No matter what you do, you can't get EVERYTHING you want to do in one day! Repeat that point until it sinks in.

_____

The important thing to remember is you don't have to lose all your Type A qualities, but you should work on ridding the unhealthy tendencies.

Now, what about the Type B personalities? Again, from looking at the chart you might think they don't experience much stress or fear. The usual view of Type B is laid back, dreamy, relaxed. However, look at the unhealthy tendencies.

The unhealthy Type B hesitates, or in another word, procrastinates. Nothing causes more stress, anxiousness, and fear than procrastination. For instance, the boss gives you a project that has to be done in three days.

Well if you are unsure of yourself, hesitant, have a low self-esteem, how are you realistically going to do that? That lack of confidence will lead to a fear of failing the task, or not getting it turned in on time.

Note in the healthy Type B, there is confidence, an awareness of time, and generally, they will be less likely to hurry and make sure that the task is accomplished correctly and turned in on time.

Therefore, whether you are a Type A or B, or a mix of the two, the goal is to try to eliminate the unhealthy or negative qualities of each, and "BALANCE" so that you can cope with the duties, stressors you face without anxiety or fear.

Another set of personality types we have to look at are whether or not we are an **EXTERNALIZER** or an **INTERNALIZER**.

What determines which one we are is how we assign or accept the responsibility for the things that happen in our life depends on which type.

If we live by the belief that it is luck and chance that are the ruling factors of whether or not we are happy, then we are living our life as an internalizer.

If on the other hand, we believe that if we want a happy life and that to get there means that we have to work hard for it, then we are an externalizer.

The following questions will help you to decide

which one you are.

1. Are most unhappy events in your life the result of bad luck or because of your mistakes?

2. Does it pay to prepare a lot for tests, or is it impossible to study for most tests?

3. Can ordinary people influence the government, or do a few people in power run things?

4. Do good friendships just happen because the chemistry is right, or do friendships happen because both people are making attempts to get along?

4. Does it pay to plan things out in detail, or do you believe that most things just work out as a matter of good or bad fortune anyhow?

5. Do you believe that what happens to you mostly your own doing (mistakes), or are most things beyond your control?

If you believe in fate or luck, chemistry or fortune, you are an externalizer. If you believe you are the captain of your soul, you are an internalizer.

Why would it be better to be an internalizer than an externalizer? Simple. When it comes to stress, anxiety, and fear, you are less likely to experience it if you take charge of your own life and not leave it up to chance, or the stars, but to your own self-determination and will.

The truth is that there are no good days or bad days. The Sun rises and falls, and "life happens" day after day. It is how YOU perceive the situations you face. Yet YOU are in control of YOUR response. True there are less than desirable things that happen to us from time to time. However, they do not control how we feel or how we act. Only we can determine that for ourselves.

CHAPTER SIX EXERCISE

Question 1: Which personality type do you see yourself as, Type A, B, or a mix? Additionally, where can you see what personality type you identify with has a direct relationship to your level of stress, anxiety and fear?

_____

_____

_____

_____

Question 2: What changes do you see in your self-identified personality type you can make to lessen your reaction to stress, anxiety and fear?

CHAPTER 6 – WHAT KIND OF PERSONALITY ARE YOU

_____

_____

_____

_____

_____

_____

_____

_____

_____

_____

_____

_____

Question 3: Do you see yourself as an

Internalizer or an Externalizer? Why and how

do you think you can change your beliefs and

how you cope with stress, anxiety and fear?

_____

_____

_____

_____

_____

_____

_____

_____

CHAPTER 7 - COPING WITH STRESS, ANXIETY & FEAR

We've now come to the final couple of chapters of this book on coping with stress, anxiety, and fear. So far, we've seen that stress, anxiety, and fear come mostly from the way we view life and the things that happen in it.

We've seen how our thinking directly affects how we feel and that determines our behavior. Now we pull the threads together and put together something we can work on to help us live without unnecessary negative stress, anxiety, and fear.

CONTROL CATASTROPHIC THINKING

Let's recap Catastrophic Thinking to make sure we understand it. If there's anything that will add to the stress, anxiety, and fear of a situation, it's making a mountain out of a molehill. For instance, have you ever had difficulty with the first item on a test and became convinced that you were going to fail the whole thing?

How about when you've had a fight with your spouse and convinced yourself that the whole day is shot. Or, if you've had a toothache and were just convinced, you were going to die. If so, you have practiced Catastrophic Thinking.

Remember Catastrophic Thinking is subjective thinking gone extreme. Subjective thinking is based on PROJECTION about the future and yet unknown events. This kind of thinking is based on self-talk, where you create a greater more morbid reality than really exists.

The problem with catastrophic thinking is that it really complicates the already agitated state of the mind in the Alarm Reaction. You are already at full speed, reacting to real events. No problem there, but add to it catastrophic thinking producing fantasy situations and you can quickly lose control of your emotions and your actions. However, remember also that you can experience the Alarm Reaction to events your mind thinks is happening, which may be real or not. This is critically important to remember.

The way that you control catastrophic thinking is with thoughts that are incompatible with it. For instance, instead of saying, "Oh my god, I can't deal with losing my wallet right now!" you say, "Ok, take a breath; it's not the end of the world."

When you think about it for a minute, it's really not. You tell yourself (self-talk), that it has to be somewhere in the house, or ask yourself, "Ok, calm down, where is the last place I saw it." Give yourself a break we all lose things. After a while, if you can't find it, then you can go and check the status of your money with the bank, credit card places, etc. Yeah, it will be a hassle to get all those cards stopped and replace your driver's license, but you don't have to lose your mind about it. What good will that really do? As I've found out when I simply calm myself and keep it real and in the now, my wallet, keys, whatever, simply shows up! Amazing how that works, but it's really not hard to understand. When you are in an agitated (fight or flight) state your mind simply cannot analyze what is going on.

Then you use incompatible thoughts to combat catastrophic thinking, it makes you accurately assess the actual situation that is happening. This keeps subjective thinking to a minimum. Remember too, that catastrophic thinking is also negative thinking. To counteract a negative thought you have to think positive counter-thoughts. "It's OK, I find it!"

At first, this isn't easy, but you didn't learn the habit of negative thinking overnight. To change a habit it takes repetition of a replacement habit. Along these lines, if you want to become an internalizer instead of an externalizer you are going to have to control subjective thinking.

You do this by staying in the NOW and not PROJECTING what might happen. Combat those subjective negative thoughts with incompatible objective positive thoughts.

So bringing those catastrophic thoughts down a couple of notches, will also reduce the stress, the anxiety, and the fear as well.

GET A HANDLE ON AUTOMATIC

THOUGHTS

You really can't do much about automatic thoughts, but you can sweep away the NAT's, the Negative Automatic Thoughts. The way to do this is, in the beginning, is to catch those NAT's on paper, and see the thought/emotion connection. In other words, asking, "Where is this thought leading me?" Negative thoughts mean negative emotions that lead to negative stress, anxiety, and fear.

Using the cases of the car keys, your child lost in the store, the near accident, the initial thoughts were negative. That is your mind went immediately to the negative.

In all cases, you could have taken things differently, thinking the event with calmer thoughts, and so calmer emotions, which lead to a positive reaction.

THE CAR KEYS

Instead of thinking "Oh no, I'm going to be late for work and get fired!" think instead, "Oh well, I guess I didn't put them where I could find them." "I'll give it a few minutes to find them, then perhaps call into work and tell them I'm running late." You would be amazed how just that phone call will calm you down.

CHILD LOST IN THE STORE

This might prove much more difficult especially in

the light of the awful things that happen today, nevertheless, you could think instead, "Ok, concentrate, where was the last place I saw them? "Ok, let me go to the Customer Service/Security desk and let them know I can't find my child."

You can see that is a much more rational and positive thought process than running around in circles thinking the worst.

NEAR MISS ACCIDENT

Although the near miss might scare you, "Omg, he almost hit me!" You can catch your thoughts and say, "Well, that was close, I so thankful it wasn't an accident, oh well, and I'm not going to let it ruin my day, accidents happen" and go ahead and drive on your way.

Again, instead of a negative thought process, you turn it into a positive and thankful thought process. In fact, if it happened on the day you were delayed by the car keys, how do you know that delay didn't save you from actually getting into the accident?

You don't, but you would be surprised at what we avoid just by a split second.

In all these cases, the thinking is first, whether you chose the negative or the positive. However, think through the ABCs and ask, is the consequence worth it.

Remember also how also negative stress can negatively affect your health and wellbeing.

One exercise I used in my stress class factored in the

EVENT vs. THE RESPONSE

Many times our response level is way too high to the level of the incident. For instance, consider that an asteroid is heading towards earth that will extinguish all life as being a 10 on the list of events that could happen today.

Now think of having a stress reaction (fear and anxiety) based on a 10 being the worst and breaking a shoelace being a 1.

Then using our examples, for instance, the near car

accident. Let's call that the 2nd level on our event list, yet you take your response to a 10th level.

It would be a little bit overkill, wouldn't it? However, we do that every day. All because of negative thinking, "Oh my goodness the world is over." (That would be real IF the asteroid is really coming, btw, but it's not), you think, "No, it's not, I just missed an accident."

Like a toothache, you could think, "I'm dying!" However, how about thinking, "No, I just have a toothache. Yeah, it hurts, but it's likely not going to kill me. I'll just go to the Dentist and get it fixed".

So constantly checking our thoughts, making sure our first thought isn't a negative, replacing it with a positive one, and rationally matching the importance to the level of the event will go a long way to reducing our stress and so our anxiety and fear.

It's not really hard to turn negative thoughts into the habit of positive ones. Habit comes from repetition so the more you practice the better you get at it. Remember how practice makes better, and not perfect?

We will not ever get perfect at it, but over time, we will at least know when we take the negative, we know what is happening.

LEARNING TO GEAR DOWN – WATCHING YOUR STRESS CUE

The diagram on the next page resembles a

speedometer. The range on the meter is from

"Slow" to "Whoa!"

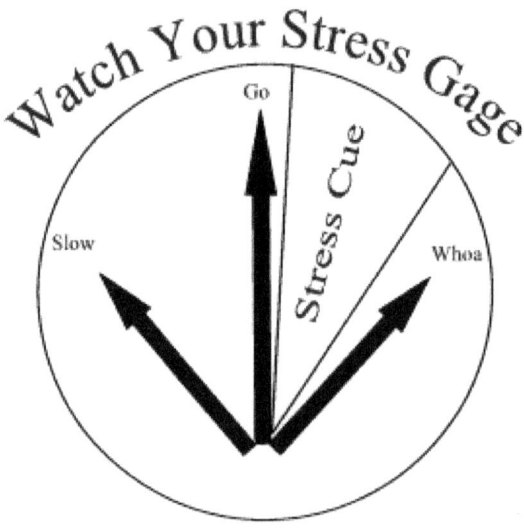

The "trick" here is to recognize your particular cue.

The cue is when you first realize that your body is

beginning to "race". As you can see, there is no real

problem in the "Slow" or "Go" mode. In fact, it is

good to be in the "Go" mode because that's where we do our best work.

However, we have the tendency to "over-rev" our engines, and you can sense when this is taking place.

For instance, you may find it difficult to catch your breath. You can feel your heart racing. On the other hand, perhaps it's a cognitive example, such as snapping at someone. Or, it could be cursing under your breath. Whatever it is, it's your "cue" to "back off the accelerator", and slow down. So as an example.

To determine your stress cue ask yourself:

I usually over-react when,

_____

_____

_____

I know something is getting to me when,

_____

_____

_____

Therefore my stress cue is,

_____

_____

_____

By learning and practicing effective coping

techniques, you can "de-accelerate" and bring

yourself off the "red line".

CHAPTER SEVEN EXERCISE

Question 1: Give an example that has happened to you more than once where you know you've overreacted. Then using what you've learned here, explain how you plan to approach that same or similar situation in the future to reduce the negative stress, anxiety and fear.

_____

_____

_____

_____

_____

CHAPTER 7 - COPING WITH STRESS, ANXIETY & FEAR

CHAPTER EIGHT – NEGATIVE & POSITIVE COPING TOOLS

We've seen that in our thinking, beliefs about events, we can have errors that complicate our process of coping.

We can't change the stressful nature of the world or control people, places, and things. However, we can learn how to cope with the pressures on us. We can do this by learning to manage our reactions to our environment, and the demands it places on us.

Coping isn't hard. Just as there is negative and positive stress, there are negative and positive coping tools. All too often, we use the negative coping methods we have learned through life. These are known as "Defensive Coping Mechanisms".

DEFENSIVE COPING

We have all used Defensive Coping Mechanisms to deal with stress. The problem with defensive coping is that while they reduce the immediate impact of the stressor, they do so at a cost to the individual. Let's look at some of these mechanisms in detail

AGGRESSION

You get cut off in traffic. You get mad and tailgate the guy for five miles, honking your horn and giving them a rather familiar hand gesture. In the meantime, you're driving recklessly and are putting yourself in danger. Punching your nutty boss in the nose gives you relief from his tyranny, but you might be looking for a job tomorrow. Aggression is a very common way that many people deal with stress. It's not always a negative way of dealing with stress, as in the case of an actual physical attack on your person you would be in your right to defend yourself.

However, when the attack is minimal or even non-existent aggression can be detrimental. Moreover, the aggressive behavior most always heightens the arousal (puts the pedal to the metal), and so heightens the conflict.

REGRESSION

You don't get your way. An obstacle frustrates your goal. Therefore, you throw a temper tantrum. You yell and scream and "turn blue" until you get your way. This might work for a 6-year old. However, when you're thirty-two, it's called regression. It means that when under conflict, pain, anxiety, we return to a former behavior characteristic of a younger age of development.

WITHDRAWAL

Whenever the stress of life is too great for us to cope with, we withdrawal either physically or psychologically. Sometimes a withdrawal of short duration can afford us the time to find some time to rest and reflect. However, when withdrawal becomes the habit or prolonged it can become a problem.

DENIAL

Some people cope with stress by denying the danger altogether.   In fact, terminally ill patients in the first stage of their diagnosis deny they are going to die. When people deny as a response to bad news, "I don't want to hear it", is a form of denial. Or they shy away from anything negative thinking, "Our of sight, out of mind, so it's not real!" However, denial doesn't change the reality of the situation nor afford any solution to the problem that is presented in it.

Denial is simply lying to yourself about what is the reality. In fact, you could say denial stands for Don't Even Know I'm Lying!

SUPPRESSION

When you consciously and purposely put stressful things out of your mind in order to avoid dealing with them, you are suppressing them. For instance, you get a notice from the IRS and you shove it in a drawer, "I'll deal with it later…" You say. You walk away and get your mind on something else. That's suppression, as well as a bit of denial

DISPLACEMENT

Your spouse argues with you before you to work.

When you get to work, you take it out on your co-workers. This is where the expression, "Kick the dog", comes from. When we displace we don't confront the stressor, we stuff the emotion and it comes out against someone or something else.

RATIONALIZATION

Rationalization is explaining away unacceptable behavior in order to exonerate ourselves.

This is the way that we cut our losses; explain away our failures, or when things don't go right. We use it to eat ice cream when we're on a diet. Pick up a cigarette when we are trying to quit smoking, and, use excuses like, "Hey, I'm sorry I yelled at you, I was just tired." Rationalization places the blame for our behavior on something or someone else. When we rationalize, we can place the blame on anyone but ourselves.

WHY DEFENSIVE COPING DOESN'T WORK!

Defensive coping methods may give us a temporary "break" from the stressor, but they do not solve the conflict or deal directly with the stressor. We cannot fix or manipulate people, places and things to fit our "liking". If we are going to deal with stress, we are going to have to do it directly with Active Coping.

ACTIVE COPING

Active coping involves taking responsibility for your life and for your response to it. Instead of using aggression, regression, withdrawal, denial, repression, displacement and rationalization to cope with life, rather than use self-deception, we **<u>ACTIVELY AND FIRMLY</u>** address with the stress in our life. If we are unhappy with our lives and the about the things that are happening to us, then WE have to take charge of our lives in order to change our life.

<u>MEDITATION</u>

When we picture meditation, we usually see a levitating Yogi, lost in a trance. Well, that is one form of meditation. However, meditation at its simplest essence is simply taking time out to put your mind at ease by concentrating on a more peaceful and serene situation. It's taking your mind off of "things" for a while, and putting them somewhere else. Now, this isn't possible during an emergency call, but when you get a break, or a little time out, go somewhere quiet, sit back, close your eyes, and think of something peaceful. Put your mind on something like your children, or revisit your honeymoon. Actually, you meditate every day and likely don't know it. That is when you daydream. It's the same thing. You can do it during a traffic jam (but please not while driving). Instead of pounding the steering wheel, cursing the delay, think about something you like, or about what you are going to

do this weekend.

PROGRESSIVE RELAXATION

Pick a muscle, any muscle and contract it as tight as

you can. Hold it for about ten seconds and then

release. This is progressive relaxation. This

decreases the tension in the muscles, which comes as

a result of the Alarm Reaction. It is most effective if

you do it at the onset of the Alarm Reaction.

DIAPHRAGMIC BREATHING

When you were a baby, you breathed correctly. That

is, you breathed from your diaphragm. If you watch

a baby breathe, you will see their stomach rise and

fall. As we become adults, we lose that ability and begin to breathe with our chest. Breathing this way is shallower and limits the amount of oxygen to the cells and blood. This places stress on the body. To begin to retrain your body to breath correctly, practice diaphragmatic breathing. A good way to do this is while sitting in your chair; place your hands on your stomach and breathe in slowly while watching your hands. With practice, you will be breathing like a baby before long.

CHANGE THE PACE OF YOUR LIFE

If you are a Type A go-getter, learn to modify your behavior. Confront the value system that accompanies your Type A beliefs. Do you believe in competition? Try cooperation. Do you want to achieve? Everyone does. However, realize that you can accomplish goals much better through appreciating life and others in it.

Challenge the idea that you must be perfect in all you do. Lose your fear of failure. We all fail sometimes. We're human. In actuality, the more perfect you try to be the more miserable and mistake prone you will tend to be.

Instead of jumping out of bed to an obnoxiously loud alarm clock, racing around the house and trying to get everything done by yourself, change your pace. Stop driving yourself crazy. Get up earlier and go to bed earlier. Learn to delegate to others, don't try to do everything yourself!

MODERATE EXERCISE

Exercise might be a dirty word, but it works wonders. You don't have to run a marathon, just a 20-minute walk three days a week will do. It helps to dissipate that residue energy you have stored up from work or from life.

Even walking in place or arm twirls or ANYTHING is better than doing nothing. However, make sure you are physically able to exercise. If you haven't seen a doctor in years, get a checkup.

LEARN TO MAKE POSITIVE AND

INTELLIGENT DECISIONS

Conflict is a stress producer. Whatever the conflict

you can become better at arriving at a solution by

weighing the pros and cons of a decision. On a

sheet of paper, write the name of the problem at the

top. Then list four questions:

1. Project all tangible gains and losses for yourself.
2. Project all tangible gains and losses for others.
3. Project self-approval or disapproval from yourself.
4. Project self-approval or disapproval from others.

List these items in a left column on a piece of paper.

Then head two more columns, "Positive

Anticipations" and the other "Negative

Anticipations". What this will do is give you a

picture of the situation you're facing from both angles. It takes the "What-If?" out of the picture and helps you to arrive at a well thought out decision. If you do this, long enough you'll learn to do it by heart and quickly assess pros and cons of every problem you run up against.in life.

When you become more decisive in your life, you will lessen the effects of its demands on you. You will more in control of your thoughts, emotions, and actions.

Dealing with Stress, Fear and Anxiety isn't hard; it just takes some basic tool for you to learn to help you positively cope.

The tips and information I gave you in this book will

help you do just that. However, everyone is individual in the way that they respond to stress, fear, and anxiety, and so take this information into forming your own plan of coping with them.

That's what I have done, and know you can do it too. It's my hope that this book helped you to understand stress, anxiety, and fear in your own life better, and helps you reduce their effects in your life.

Good luck and God bless.

CHAPTER EIGHT EXERCISE

Question 1: What type of coping tools have you been using before you read this book; Defensive or

Active? Have you discovered how one worked

better for you than the other, if so why?

_____

_____

_____

_____

_____

_____

_____

_____

_____

_____

_____

_____

_____

_____

_____

_____

Please visit tpmcatamney.com for more information, helpful tips. You can also reach the author at tpmac58@gmail.com for more individual help with your particular stress reduction needs.

www.ingramcontent.com/pod-product-compliance
Lightning Source LLC
Chambersburg PA
CBHW071422180526
45170CB00001B/192